# General Extra Care

# General Extra Care

*The Full Facts*

V K Leigh

| Library of Congress Control Number: | | 2012914521 |
| --- | --- | --- |
| ISBN: | Hardcover | 978-1-4771-5562-2 |
| | Softcover | 978-1-4771-5561-5 |
| | Ebook | 978-1-4771-5563-9 |

This book was printed in the United States of America.

**To order additional copies of this book, contact:**
Xlibris Corporation
0-800-644-6988
www.Xlibrispublishing.co.uk
Orders@Xlibrispublishing.co.uk
304647

# CONTENTS

# About this Book

The roles of the modern sheltered scheme manager have changed drastically. Modernisation in sheltered housing has created new rules in the field of sheltered housing and also to the modern sheltered scheme manager.

The sheltered scheme managers of today must be well mannered, cultured, educated and must be computer literate; more so are the expectations that this book brings into light the awareness behind the facts.

The roles of the modern sheltered scheme manager are more complicated than ever and there are many dos and don'ts that need to be registered in peoples' minds as this book is being read.

This book educates anyone and everyone that reads it, of the inner working procedures and abilities of the sheltered scheme managers.

This book is an educational material that can be used to train/ teach a sheltered scheme manager to be.

This book can be used as a quick reference to the duties of a sheltered scheme manager and those related to similar duties.

This book is written with intent to familiarise persons involved with the day to day services of older people.

It is also to lighten the awareness of Housing Associations, Health visitors, Social Services, Housing Organisations, National Health Services (NHS), Housing related staff, Persons with Interest of being a sheltered scheme manager.

# Acknowledgements

This book is dedicated to all those People and Organisations that understand, appreciate and know how it feels like to take care of the Older People.

I would like to appreciate my colleagues that gave me an insight to the challenges that brought about the awareness and understanding of the issues which have greatly enriched this publication.

I would like to thank my wife and children for their scrutiny, contributions and patience in times of challenges during the preparation of these materials and writing of this book.

I would like to thank God Almighty for the inspiration given to me in the times of writing and during its publication.

My gratitude goes to my wife, Fatimah, whom in her tirelessness efforts made sure that this book is produced wholly.

# Introduction

Every housing related organisation has strategic Equalities and Visions for their would-be tenants, residence and for themselves; to guide them more positively towards successful business ventures.

No individuals or groups should be at a disadvantage by reason of ethnicity, gender, sexual orientation, age, employment status and religious beliefs.

The organisation accepts that everyone has rights to their diverse identity.

The organisation understands that the valuing of diversity will improve and better the services being provided.

Through training and development, the employees are able to achieve the organisation's objectives.

The organisation provides services to the diverse needs of the communities.

When a tenant moves into an Extra Care Sheltered housing scheme, a welcoming pack is organised and given by the housing organisation. In this pack, all important and immediate valuable information including telephone numbers relating to things such as repairs, housing officer and emergencies are enclosed for the tenant's convenience.

# MISSION STATEMENT

A Mission statement is a statement of purpose characterised by that organisation.

A MISSION STATEMENT reads as follows—

- WE ARE COMMITTED TO RESPONDING TO CHANGING NEEDS, WORKING TOGETHER WITH EXTERNAL AGENCIES AND MONITORING THE NEEDS OF OUR TENANTS.

All housing organisations have their own Philosophy Underpinning the sheltered housing services that they operate, e.g. "Managing and respecting the delicate balance between observances of individual's welfare and rights also that of others.

# PERSONALISATION

Personalisation in the sheltered scheme environment means thinking about care and support services.

It starts with the person as an individual, looking at their strengths, their preferences, aspirations, identifying their needs and making choices about what, who, how and when they are supported to live their lives. It needs a significant transformation of adult social care so that all systems, processes, staff and services are geared up to put people first.

Personalisation is addressing the needs and desire of the whole communities to ensure everyone has access to the right information, advice and advocacy to make good decisions about the support they need. It means ensuring that people have wider choice in how their needs are met and are able to access universal services such as transport, leisure and education, housing, health and opportunities for employment regardless of age or disability.

The care for older persons is a complex and skilled branch of health care.

To be effective, careers need to be knowledgeable, flexible and positive in their interventions. The objectives are based on the idea that care for older people needs to be holistic. This means that in order to be effective a career must consider the client from biological, psychological and sociological viewpoints.

It is essential to underpin this holistic assessment with an insight into the relationships between the client's individual needs and the attitudes and resources that currently exist in the UK.

Housing organisations deliver wider range of services that promote independence and prevent people from needing institutional forms of care.

These include: Adaptations, Design, Flexible Ownership Options (FOO), Advice and Information, Telecare, Supported and Sheltered housing, Support Services based on individual needs such as a Handyperson services.

Personalisation hasten developments already in existence within the housing sectors especially in sheltered housing giving the people more control and choice over their living environment.

Sheltered housing is provided by the following bodies:

- Local authority—rent only
- Voluntary sector—rent only
- Housing associations—rent or part buy
- Private Organizations—buy only

In either situation, it is proper to think about the costs of the property and services charges.

## Personalisation for home care providers

*This briefing was co-produced with the United Kingdom Homecare Association Ltd (UKHCA).*

Published: June 2009

This relates to Extra Care schemes also where the residents are cared for 24hours, 7 days per week.

Personalisation for home care providers means:

- recognising that the types of support that people who use services say they need may not be confined to personal care—they can include a much wider range of tasks
- developing systems and training to enable staff to expand their skills and to work in creative, person-centred ways
- thinking about how to contribute to the expansion of the personal assistant (PA) workforce and to the increasing need for specialist services by diversifying into these markets
- recognising that home care services, whether provided directly by the council, paid for privately or by personal budget holders, must be focused on identifying and achieving outcomes
- local authorities and providers working together so that home care providers have the freedom to innovate and use budgets flexibly as agreed with the person using services.

In addition:

- capacity, recruitment and retention are increasingly important issues
- Personalisation has the potential to give home care providers a good opportunity to make work more interesting and rewarding.

Personalisation means starting with the person as an individual with strengths, preferences and aspirations and putting them at the centre of the process of identifying their needs and making choices about what, who, how and when they are supported to live their lives. It requires a significant transformation of adult social care so that all systems, processes, staff and services are geared up to put people first.

Housing providers already deliver a wide range of services that promote independence and prevent people needing more intensive and institutional forms of care. These include:

- adaptations
- inclusive design
- flexible ownership options
- advice and information

- preventative technology and Telecare
- supported and sheltered housing
- support services based on individual needs and preferences
- Handyperson and care and repair schemes.

Personalisation is about giving the people more choice and control over their lives in all social care settings and is far wider than simply giving personal budgets to people eligible for council funding.

Personalisation means addressing the needs and aspirations of the whole communities to ensure that everyone has access to the right of information, advice and advocacy and to make good decisions about the support they need.

Personalisation means ensuring that people have wider choice in how their needs are met and is able to access universal services such as transport, leisure and education, housing, health and opportunities for employment regardless of age, gender or disability.

# CARE PROVIDERS (IMPLICATIONS)—AS STATED BY "THE UNITED KINGDOM HOMECARE ASSOCIATION LTD (UKHCA)"

Care providers range from small single organisations to very large companies which provide a range of other services; all in similar style.

The impact of personalisation will be very different for organisations that have relied mainly on large-scale, council contracts compared those that have focused more on self-funding customers.

Local authorities implement personalisation at different levels, so this document should be considered in relation to the organisation concerned.

Firstly, know how this system is meant to work and then, what the process will be:

## *The Process*

Individuals can now undertake self assessment, with help from family or friends, the council, or a variety of other sources including brokers or advocates. Following this the 'indicative budget' is worked out and shared with the individual. The FACS (Fair Access to Care Services) system will still be the basis for determining eligibility for public funding, and a RAS (Resource Allocation System) is also being developed by most authorities to determine the size of personal budgets.

# WHAT IS EXTRA CARE?

Extra Care is a service that is provided for people who are unable to support themselves by living independently in their own homes even with some support.

Extra Care provides different kinds of services to different individuals with various needs.

The client group that live in Extra Care Housing Facilities are ordinary day to day people like everyone else except that they have been assessed and qualified to be given additional support in their own homes.

These services vary from intensive emergency care to helping the individual complete benefit forms and paperwork in confidence.

## What is Housing with Care?

This is all forms of specialist housing for older people where care services are provided; such as Standard Sheltered Housing, Extra Care sheltered housing and Care villages

## Extra Care Housing

Extra Care Housing is a specialised kind of sheltered housing with more demands in its management style which helps older people to maintain their independence.

Extra Care Housing is a type of Sheltered Housing that offers Care and Support

Extra Care Housing is usually managed by the Sheltered Housing Manager.

The purpose of providing Extra Care housing is to **promote** Independence—providing self contained accommodation, enabling the individual to continue to live in the community to avoid being isolated.

**Empowering** the tenant; making health, care and support services available to the individual where they live, than having to move into a residential care type of home.

It provides **accessibility** with the specially designed or adapted accommodation, facilitating the delivery of care. These care and support services are tailored to meet the individual needs of the tenants.

The sheltered scheme manager is fully responsible for the management of the scheme allocated by the organisation to his/her charge.

The sheltered scheme manager is responsible for the health and safety of everyone that is within the said scheme at anytime.

The sheltered scheme manager is the first point of contact in any sheltered accommodation.

The scheme manager or care co-ordinator is the responsible person who cares for the welfare of the tenants, the tenants' health and safety of that particular scheme.

The scheme manager and Care Coordinator are responsible for monitoring care packages, liaising with the social services and care agencies in order to ensure that the concerned individual(s) gets continuous positive service(s).

In the Extra Care environment, Scheme Manager is assisted by the Care Coordinator who is in charge of the Carers and makes an impact to the care being rendered to the tenants living in that facility.

The sheltered scheme manager is not a messenger or a door person in any scheme.

It is the duty of a scheme manager to visit the tenants or give them calls on daily basis. It is more so if the tenant is known to be vulnerable.

The scheme manager is responsible for updating the personal information on tenants' files and if for any reason(s) the tenant should need referral; then, this must be done without delays.

The scheme manager can make referrals to professional organisations on behalf of the tenants but only with the tenant's / family consent.

The scheme manager is responsible for coordinating and hosting meetings within the scheme.

The scheme manger's roles are subject to review annually by the Organisation's housing services manager.

# APPLYING FOR EXTRA CARE HOUSING

The flats and accommodations of Extra Care Housing are allocated on the outcome of the assessment carried out on the individual applicant.

This should be done in accordance with the organisation's Fair Access to Care Services and Access Criteria for this type of accommodation.

Following a referral, sometimes from the Sheltered Scheme Manager of the sheltered housing accommodation where the proposed tenant may be living at the time, the Adult and Community Services (Social Services) Care Manager will arrange to visit the proposed tenant in order to assess their needs for this type of accommodation.

Extra Care Housing supports people to live independently.

The schemes consist of self-contained flats, designed to suit the needs of older people.

A Sheltered Scheme Manager, Care Coordinator and Care Staff are based on site 24 hours a day to support the needs of the residents.

Extra Care Housing gives you security and privacy within your own home.

Extra Care Housing is **housing** with care and support for older people

There are some benefits that also come with living in Extra Care sheltered housing.

## *Vulnerable Tenants*

The vast majority of vulnerable tenants in extra-care sheltered schemes are supported by social services, family members and vetted friends; through the hospital when they become ill and monitored by the scheme manager.

The scheme manager makes referral to the social services by alerting them of the tenant's needs either from information received when writing the support plans or discussion with the tenant but with the tenant's knowledge.

The social service then carries out an agreed assessment which will provide the individual with a suitable Care package that allows them to live an independent lifestyle as best as possible.

# BENEFITS

Care staffs are rota based and made available 24 /7 to provide care and support.

In some Organization, the Rota based staff plays important role while visiting carers are not on scene.

The staffs provide morning and evening calls/ visits.

The staff will assist with letters, bills and filling of official forms for the tenants.

The staff will assist where a carer might be running late; if/when laundry for the tenant is incomplete but can only do so when informed by the carer.

The staffs are likely to assist with toileting between carer's calls.

There is security and privacy with each tenant's own front door making the tenant to decide whom you let into your house or not.

Each tenant will sign a legal tenancy agreement between them and the housing authority/association.

Couples stay together as they should in their own home

You have self control over your finances.

There are full programmes of activities.

You are living at home—not in a home!

Extra Care housing is a very exciting project to be developed for the older people in different parts of the world especially in the UK; where the ageing population the ageing population and the rest of the world are increasing fast.

Survey shows that the older population will be doubled in the next ten to twenty years.

The older and vulnerable persons will experience deterioration in their health and will definitely need support in order to live their lives more fully.

Extra Care housing is a place that will help the tenants with continuity of their life styles with independence and security is called Extra Care sheltered housing.

Extra Care offers people the opportunity to live independently in a home of their own; whether they have low or high support needs, it makes no difference. Some services include offers such as social activities and learning opportunities.

In the Sheltered and Extra Care Housing industries, there are always waiting lists.

Sheltered housing should not be mistaken for Extra Care housing and vice versa.

Sheltered housing is for people that are able to manage with little or no assistance; this, in comparison to Extra Care Housing where they are purpose built to enable specialist assistance from external organisation. This allows freedom and independence no matter how bad the situation may be.

## People in Extra Care Type of Housing

These are people who have been assessed and qualified to be given extra supports while in a care home or in their own homes.

These are people readily assessed but with lesser needs compared to the people who are living in residential care homes.

Extra Care Housing provides a range of housing and care/support services tailored to meet individual needs available 24 hours a day, 7 days a week.

The amount of care provided at any time should be flexible to accommodate fluctuating needs where some tenants could be away to hospitals, Day Centres. This is a supported service by in-built "smart technology" or Community Alarm Services is commonly known (an alarm system used to alert staff in emergencies).

Extra Care Sheltered Housing Schemes are designed to cater for specialist needs, such as for people with dementia, wheelchair users etc. Living within a supervised community can help some people to maintain and build up the skills needed to retain their independence.

Supported housing as is commonly called, is available to people with a wide range of support needs, for example:

- Older people with physical difficulties
- Older people with special needs.
- Older people who need support to manage their own homes.
- Older people with mental health needs
- Older people with learning difficulties

Extra Care Sheltered Housing Schemes could be regarded as a small community of its own that provides care to its tenants; which could be in the sheltered homes or in their own private homes.

This Extra Care Homes become the homes of these tenants for the rest of their lives except when they decide to move to a different place of accommodation. Then a transfer is put into place.

Tenants live as independent individuals and as time passes by each one gets older and may need extra package of care for a better living condition with the help of the care staff; this is made a reality.

Extra Care accommodations are purpose built to accommodate the everyday need of each tenant.

Each flat is fitted with smoke alarm.

Some of the purpose built Extra Care Accommodations have parking facilities and the flats are designed to fit and suit their lifestyles.

Emergency intercom alarm system is available in each flat.

When ever assistance is needed anywhere in your home or garden, press the red button on the pendant worn round the neck or wrist watch-like pendant on your wrist.

The operator immediately responds by speaking through the "Smart Technology" equipment fitted in the flat asking if all is well and if not, what the problem could be what kind of help is needed and will then act accordingly.

The lightweight pendant is easy to wear round the neck, like wearing a necklace or could be worn round the wrist as a wrist watch.

The other option could be by pulling the pull cords installed in each room in the flat including the toilets and bathrooms/ walk-in shower rooms.

No other special kind of equipment will be needed. There are two types of equipment presently;

## Telecare—Emergency Team

Telecare—emergency team—is a 24 hour communication service primarily for the elderly, disabled or other vulnerable people enabling them to remain living independently in their own home in any area of the country. Their service is available to tenants in sheltered and general housing, as well as owner-occupiers.

Telecare offers you the reassurance of knowing that in an emergency or serious difficulty, help can be summoned 24 hours a day and 365 days a year at the press of a button or by pulling the emergency cords in the accommodation.

There is always an immediate response guaranteed, no matter what the situation may be. The response is determined by the nature of the problem. The skilled staff at the Control Centre can alert the emergency services (Fire, Police or Ambulance) contact a personal carer, a nominated friend or relative, or send a mobile warden out to your home.

You are given the feel of safety assurance at the end of the phone.

# EMERGENCY EQUIPMENT

## Dispersed Alarm-

**This** is an old time gadget that is still in use by some organisations, especially, Local Government housing organisations. This is plugged into an electronic socket, together with an existing landline telephone, inclusive, a pendant that comes in the kit.

## Scheme Pendant

This is a programmed pendant by the sheltered scheme manager which takes only a few minutes to set up. It is worn round the neck in the form of a necklace and can also be worn as a wrist watch round the wrist.

The later, being more adaptable to work directly with the pull cords relating to each flat involved.

It has also been known that some dispersed alarm pendants can be programmed to work in some of the extra-care sheltered schemes, connected with pull cords; but more directly to the call centre as a direct link in emergencies.

## Functions of the Pendants/Pull Cords

Important functions of the pendants/pull cords are to summon help automatically and immediately by dialling the help line on behalf of the individual whenever an assistant is needed.

When the individual presses the red button or pulls the strings to the pull cords in the flat; an immediate response is received at the call centre; the person involved can then respond from anywhere within the flat, without going over to the phone or installed equipment. Sometimes the person involved could just press the red button on the pendant and talk to the operator from the comfort of their chair/bed and assistance will be arranged immediately. Occasionally, the person may need assistance outside their flats when in the communal areas. There are call points available in the communal areas that enable two-ways communications to be made.

# THE VEGA—AV3

This wrist-watch like gadget is modern and highly recommended especially for those tenants who wander about unknowingly.

This is known as the **"safety walking watch";** with technology improving, these are locators in the form of a wrist watch. It is known as "The Vega—AV3—The Safety Walking Watch".

It comes very useful to locate people with dementia that wander about without knowing where they might be. It makes identification easier for the police when found. Family member can speak to the individual through it. It has a red button that can be pushed on its side to make it become as a pendant; in times of an emergency, to call for help. It uses similar signal as a mobile phone.

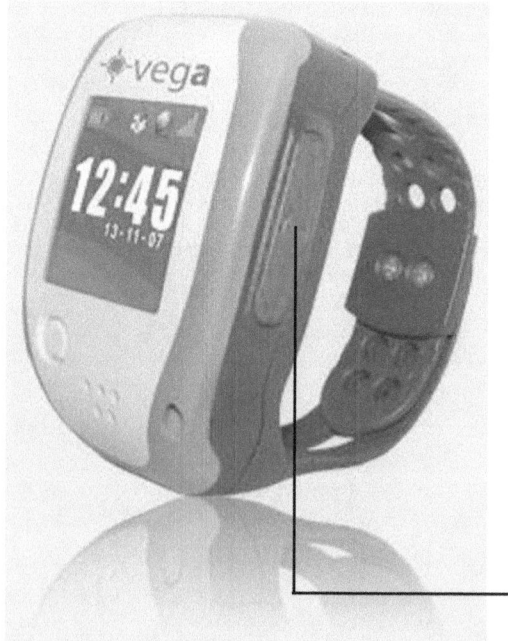

➤**Press to call**

# COSTS

The costs of the accommodation vary from place to place and from one organisation to another.

An approximate figure could be:

An outright sale of £130,000 plus.

Shared ownership between the tenant/owner and the housing organisation could be from £65,000 plus.

Renting—The rent can be from £110.00 per week which includes ground rent and most of the facilities such as heating, laundry facility, etc.

There are five things that need to be considered where costs for renting a flat in the Extra Care sheltered accommodation.

The Extra Care sheltered housing is not for free; like any other housing, *rent* need to be charged—Housing Benefit is applicable depending on the tenant's incoming finance.

*Care Costs* are charged—assistance may be available through the Social Services depending on the income.

*Support Costs* are charged but if on housing benefit, it becomes a waiver.

***Service charges*** are linked with the home such as calling in for repairs when there is a pipe leakage in the flat or in the communal area such as the laundry machines—housing benefit is a possibility.

The ***tenant is responsible for all the other services*** including domestics, shopping and cost of frozen meals.

# PURCHASE OF SHELTERED ACCOMMODATION

Some housing associations have leasehold sheltered accommodation within some boroughs to purchase. These properties are mainly one bedroom self-contained departments with a resident sheltered scheme manager. Applications to purchase are made to the housing association / agent.

The condition is that you must be 60 plus to qualify and should be able to purchase outright or part purchase in some schemes.

There is an additional service charge; which cover the cost of general maintenance, cleaning buildings, insurance etc.

There is usually a waiting list for these properties and the association will normally contact applicants when a property becomes available.

Each property is fully equipped with the "smart technology" equipments and fit to function as an Extra Care accommodation.

## Rental of Extra Care Sheltered Accommodation

These flats are purpose built for wheel chair access, usually part-furnished and are rented the same way as a normal council housing. The exception is that you do not have the right to buy them.

Sheltered housing must not be confused with Residential Care Homes; although care needs are provided to some tenants who tend to confuse the outsiders even some professionals.

Care is provided for some of its people that suffer from learning difficulties or mental illness.

Sheltered housing schemes are not 'old peoples' homes' neither are they residential care homes; although Extra Care facilities may be available and provided, it is still a place that can be called home with some independence attached to it.

Sheltered Housing gives people the opportunity to live in a community with people of similar age group while retaining their independence.

Sheltered housing is aimed at older people who are independent and able to manage alone for most of the time but prefer the added security of an alarm call system and care; thereby the Extra Care facilities. Scheme Mangers visit and make contacts with all tenants of sheltered housing every working day, as required, to ascertain their welfare and to see if there are matters in which they could provide support or advice. Tenants of sheltered housing and Extra Care sheltered Housing are independent and capable of undertaking most of their own household activities.

Sheltered housing is a positive option for older people.

It does not solve the problems of isolation and loneliness, particularly if this is caused by a wish not to mix socially.

This should not be seen as a solution to the problems of relatives.

The schemes described as extra care sheltered housing have the following features:

- Scheme Manager, project housing officer or support staff.
- Pull-cords in each room to alert the help of the scheme manager or project housing officer in an emergency; and a two-way intercom facility to speak with the Scheme Manager
- Communal Lounge
- Laundry facilities.
- Guest flat.
- Communal restaurant that is fully equipped.

- Library and IT room.
- Fitness room.
- Hairdressing room
- First aid room.
- Gardening (in some schemes)
- Wheelchair and scooter storage/garage.

Every extra care sheltered scheme building have a fitted lift, fully maintained with a maximum of two hours response call, should there be any reported faults except the bungalow type of buildings.

Ranges of activity are available and open to tenants and family members and people in the community.

There is a long list of applicants' waiting list for people who have applied for Extra Care housing accommodation. When an application is received, it does not mean that a guaranteed offer will automatically be made.

It is better to expand on the territory of the locations that are being applied for in order to limit the possibilities of delays and getting better choices.

Extra Care Housing is housing with care. In recent years, many models of Extra Care housing have been developed worldwide both in the public and private sectors and the effort continues

Housing with Care is an exciting addition to the range of housing and services available to older people in the UK.

With professional experience, this information will assist the housing market with Care to expand.

Continuous innovation with professionalism can involve:

- Sharing information educates everyone.
- Sharing knowledge and experience makes more of a success.
- By working towards a common goal for the public creates confidence.
- By delivering promises to the people; makes the people to have confidence in sheltered Care housing.

# SUITABILITY

## Suitable Candidate

The Extra Care Sheltered Housing Scheme is suitable for people aged 60years to 65years and over.

Disable people with care needs that have been assessed and approved by the housing organisations concerned.

Someone who is or may be in need of community care services by reason of mental or other disability, age or illness.

Care staffs are made available 24 hours a day and 7 days a week.

The charges are fixed weekly; plus a charge for the care that is being provided.

A Care Plan is written to support the needs that are being provided for the individual by the care organisation.

### Risk

An adult at risk is anyone aged 18 and over.

They are usually in need of community care services because of their disability, age or illness.

They are unable to take care of themselves.

Some of them are unable to protect themselves from harm and can be exploited by families, carers and professionals—more can be read under the section of abuse later.

Adults at risk can be classified as:-

- Older people with physical disabilities
- People with Mental Health.
- People with Dementia.
- Sometimes people with Ulcerated Feet do fall as victims.

# ABUSE

The above named ailments sometimes lead to violation of the individual's human and civil rights by another person(s).

They can be planned or unplanned violation.

It is called abuse and can be classified in different formats as in percentage for example, 88% of these actions could be classified as a form of abuse.

## *Types of abuse*

| | |
|---|---|
| Financial | —20% |
| Sexual | —3% (reported), 12% (unreported). |
| Physical and Emotional | —19% |
| Neglect | —12% |
| Psychological | —34% |

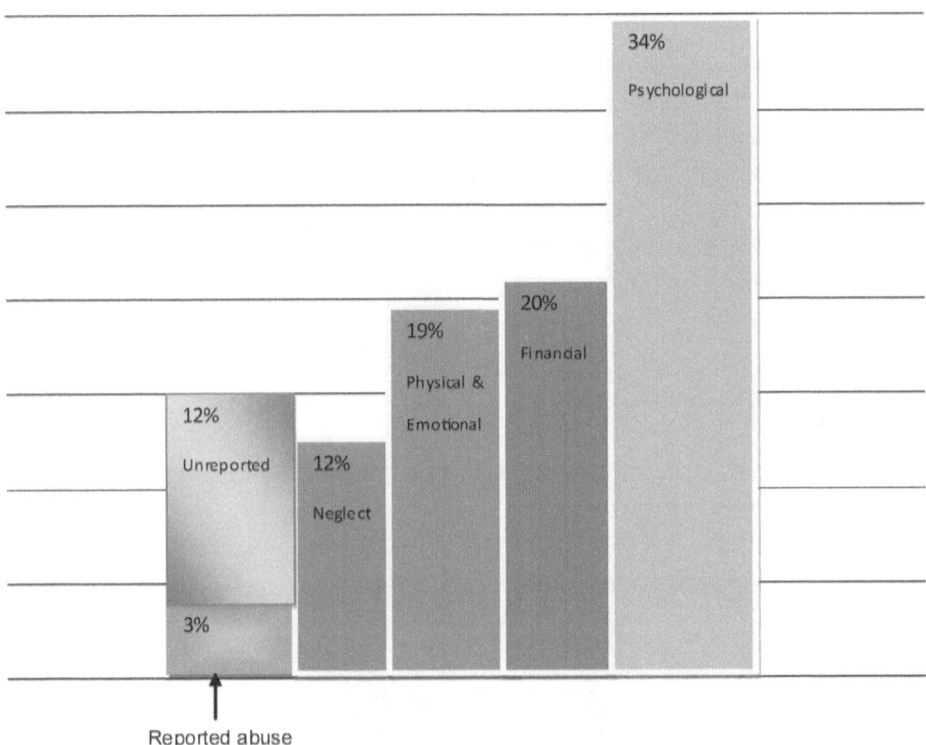

**Types of Abuse—*Diagram not to scale***

## *Financial*

This is when the person's money is being indiscriminately used, bank accounts and any other things belonging to that person.

This is the defrauding of someone's property.

## *Sexual*

Unwanted sexual activities, the touching and kissing without the consent of the person involved.

This is when someone is being forced to participate in sexual actions or conversation against their will / wishes.

## Discrimination abuse / Hate Crime.

These are other forms of harassment based on skin colour or ethnic backgrounds, racist or based on the person's disability.

This is when a person's disability and other forms of harassment or similar treatment such as racist, sexist or skin colour are being used against them.

## Physical /Emotional.

This takes the form of hitting someone, shaking also verbal abuse, bullying or being threatened.

When medication is administered inappropriately to a helpless someone

These abuses can happen in the homes or in some other places.
It can happen in residential settings.
It can happen in a day centre.
An abuse can happen in public places.

## Psychological

Threatening, using what someone loves, or values against them.

## Neglect

Not being fed (failing to provide food), heat, clothing or aids needed for survival.

## Institutional

Thank goodness for modernisations, rules and laws; this word has been ruled out from most care homes and care environment.

It used to be commonly found in any care homes or Extra Care environment.

Repeated incidents of poor practice and care that goes unaddressed

For the older people, the ages of abuse could vary; after the age of 70years, it is noted that the rate of abuses seemed to increase.

Age 55-64 years      —4%
Age 65-69 years      —18%
Age70-79 years       —22%
Age80-89 years       —40%
Age90+               —16%

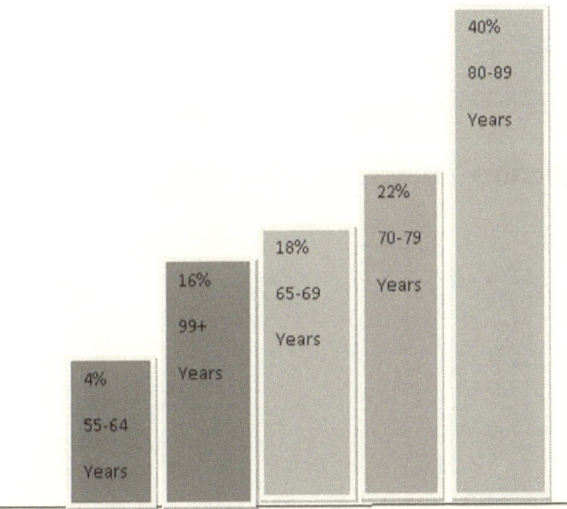

**Ages of Victims of Abuse—*diagram not to scale***

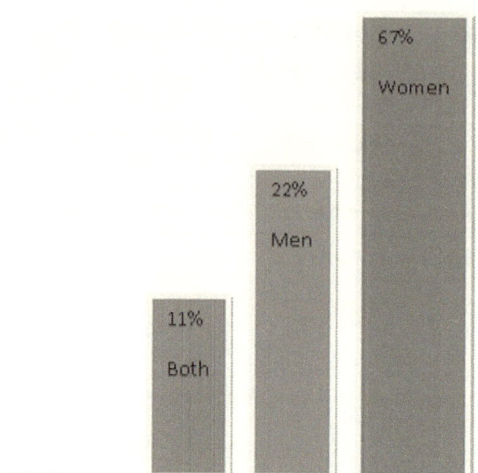

**Gender of Victims—*diagram not to scale***

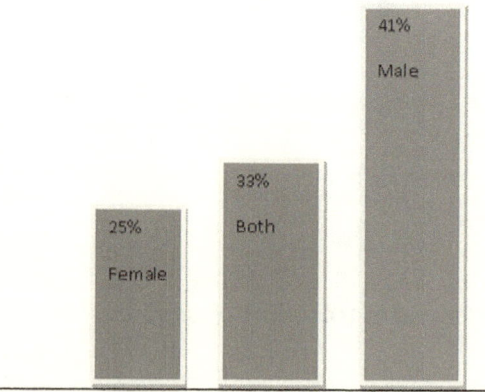

**Gender of the Abuser—*diagram not to scale***

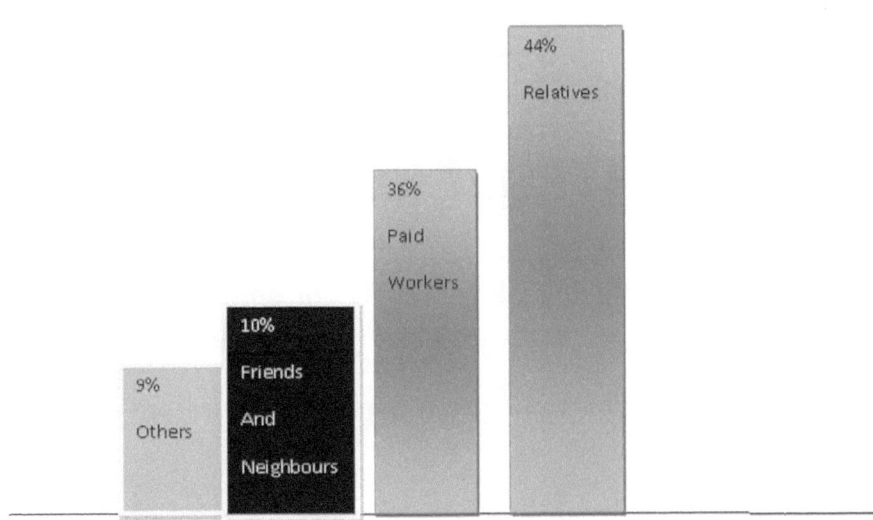

**The Abusers—*diagram not to scale***

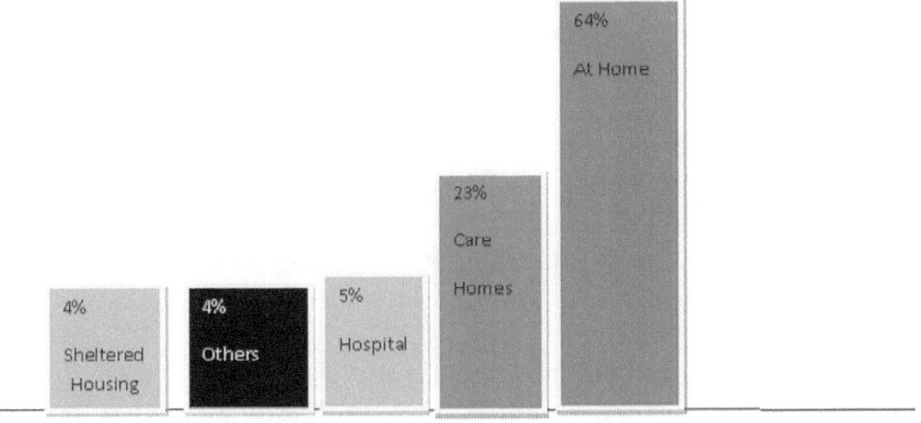

**Places Abuse commonly occur—*diagram not to scale***

# SAFEGUARDING

The oxford dictionary explains it as: proviso or other device against foreseen risks—Protection—The person who or that which guards.

Safeguarding is the act of protecting a person (Victim) from any kind of harm.

The word "safeguarding" becomes meaningful, where vulnerability is involved.

Safeguarding is a means of rendering protection to abused vulnerable victims especially in the sheltered housing and Extra Care environments; it also relates to other areas in the professional fields and in the housing environment.

There are many forms of abuse such as Emotional, Financial, Mental, Verbal, Physical and Racial, Sexual etc.

The abuse could be in the manners of being abused verbally or bullied.

In most times, the abusing person(s) are often well known to the victims. They could be a Care worker, professional worker, family member, neighbours, another tenant or an acquaintance. This is a very sensitive matter which must be reported as soon as possible to a neutral person that can alert those in authority; this matter should take a priority preference and be referred to the organisation concerned to deal with, so as not to endanger the life of the person being abused.

This is treated as a matter of confidentiality within the organisation concerned; it is handled with discretion and professionalism.

# NEW TENANTS CHECK LIST

**Name(s):** _____

**Address:** _____

**Date(s):** _____ **Completed by** _____

*Tick*

- O Introductions
- O Information Pack—Well packaged
- O Role of scheme manager / hours of work
- O Community Alarms Complete Information—System demonstration.
- O Medical Information
- O Discussion on needs—social needs / care needs / sensory needs etc.
- O Agreement on contact arrangements
- O Identify special needs
- O Social events information
- O Local information
- O Discuss how / to be called / introduced
- O Complaints / Compliments /Suggestions procedures (formal / informal).
- O Health & Safety issues
- O Security
- O Fire procedures
- O Explain Protection of Vulnerable Adult Policy
- O Laundry

- Lift
- Guest Flat
- Rubbish disposal / Recycling
- TV Licence
- Repairs reporting
- Notice Boards
- Keys
- Loop System
- Waiver Form
- Arranged Date to complete Assessment Need and Support Planning.

A convenient time can be set aside to complete the above, if there is not enough time.

An interpreter may be arranged for in exceptional cases

# CHECK LIST FOR NEW SHELTERED SCHEME MANAGER

| DAY—1 | Completed | Date |
|---|---|---|
| Introduction to tenants and scheme cleaner | | |
| **Shown Location and Use of:-** | | |
| Telecare System | | |
| Fire Alarm System | | |
| Intercom | | |
| Door Entry | | |
| CCTV—Now digital. | | |
| Keys (General) | | |
| Electricity, fuses, main switch | | |
| Lighting Controls And Emergencies | | |
| Metres | | |
| Laundry and Controls | | |
| Heating and Controls | | |
| Fire Appliances, contacts and procedures | | |
| Lifts | | |
| First Aid box | | |
| Notice Board | | |
| Guest Room | | |
| Phone Box | | |
| Kitchen | | |
| Lounge | | |

| | | |
|---|---|---|
| Refuse Areas | | |
| Smoke Detectors | | |
| Assisted Bathroom / Walk-in Shower | | |
| Loop System | | |
| *In Scheme Manager's Office* | | |
| Manual of procedures and guidance | | |
| Records of Tenants | | |
| Information on scheme | | |
| List of Emergency phone numbers | | |
| List of phone numbers | | |
| List of phone numbers of other agencies | | |
| Lists of all Scheme Managers | | |

| During First Week | Completed | Date |
|---|---|---|
| *Inside Scheme Manager's Office—DISCUSS* | | |
| Supervision / Monitoring of cleaning, Gardening, Ground Maintenance, Caretaking, Window Cleaning | | |
| Repairs Reporting | | |
| Health and safety | | |
| Risk Management | | |
| Weekly Health & Safety Scheme | | |
| Inspection Check Forms | | |
| Independent inspection | | |
| Security | | |
| Lone Working procedures | | |
| Assessment of needs and Support Planning | | |
| Contact with tenants | | |
| Complaints procedures (formal & informal) | | |
| Protection of Vulnerable Adults | | |
| Equality & Diversity | | |
| Training Records | | |

| | | |
|---|---|---|
| Support & Supervision | | |
| Other matters arising from | | |
| Manual and Exit interview with previous post holder | | |
| **End of First Week** | | |
| Service Manager interview to ensure scheme manager | | |
| Has made personal contacts with all tenants | | |
| Is familiar with all scheme facilities | | |
| Has read an understood manual | | |
| Has begun to identify objectives and tasks. | | |
| Has begun to establish contacts with other scheme managers. | | |
| Has dates of meetings and supervision in dairy | | |
| Is aware of training opportunities | | |

| | | |
|---|---|---|
| **By end of 2nd Week** | | |
| Visited central office and staff. | | |
| Is following induction programme | | |
| Has registered for appropriate training. | | |

**NAME OF SCHEME MANAGER:** _____

**NAME OF SERVICE/ OPERATION MANAGER:** _____

# STAFF TRAINING

Training is always available to staff working in the Extra Care sectors.

The staffs that work in Extra Care environment are given good opportunities to train in different courses which relate to their everyday work in areas such as-

- Moving & Handling.
- Infection Control.
- Catheter Care.
- The Prompting and Administering of Medication (PAM).
- Communication Skills.
- Emergency First Aid.
- Food Hygiene and more.

All the above training courses are vital to this industry.

The local Council' Environmental Health Officers are required by Law to carry out food hygiene inspections of All food premises in the Local borough within a period of six months and the Extra Care Kitchens are no exception.

To ensure food safe production, it will be expected to identify all steps in the activities which are critical to food safety. (Food Safety Regulations 1995, Regulation 4(3).

Ensure that adequate safety controls are in place, and that these controls are maintained and reviewed. (Food Safety Regulation 1995, Reg. 4(3))

Ensure that all staff who handles food in the place of business has undergone adequate food hygiene training or instruction according to their involvement in the food business. (Food Safety Regulations 1995, Reg. 4(2) (d).

# LONE WORKING PROCEDURES

In Extra Care sheltered housing, this may not apply because of it's a 24/7care home with staff and its operational facilities.

As a guide to the safety and welfare of the Scheme Manager,

"Lone Working Guidance Procedures" were still put in place for Health and Safety purpose and promoting safer working conditions.

## *Guidance Notes*

The guidance note is to promote safer working environment for all sheltered scheme managers when:

- -Visiting tenants in their homes.
- -Working in the communal areas of a sheltered scheme.
- -In hazardous conditions / environment.
- -Sharing tenants' information.
- -Covering other sheltered schemes.
- -Meeting with the tenants'.
- -Dealing with tenants' complaints.
- -Keeping records on the daily occurrences for tenants and the sheltered scheme.
- -End of the working day.

# HEALTH & SAFETY

## *What is Health and Safety?*

**Health** and **safety** is a cross-disciplinary area and the legal system concerned with protecting the **safety**, **health** and welfare of people engaged in work or employment.

Scheme Managers are expected to be quick on decision makings and able to defend their decisions on actions taken.

Health and Safety checks are carried out daily, in the internal and external areas of the building.

Health and Safety checks are carried out daily on all the fire extinguishers and fire signs are checked in the communal areas in order to affirm that they have not been tampered with.

The paladin bins areas are also checked to make sure that they are clean, avoiding the invitation to foxes and the infestation of mice.

There could be spillage of oil, broken bottles or water on the floor in the communal areas of the corridors.

It is also the responsibility of the sheltered scheme manager to know what kind of chemicals that the cleaners use to clean the scheme; some tenants may be allergic to some of the chemicals being used in the communal areas.

In the Extra Care buildings there are communal facilities such as fridge and freezers. These are monitored and temperature controlled on daily basis and the foods stored in them are also checked to make sure that they are still in date.

Whenever temperatures are checked, they are recorded on a special form which is then checked and if any problems, these are followed up by the Manager of the Extra Care scheme.

**Name of Shelter** _____

| Date | | | | | | |
|---|---|---|---|---|---|---|
| Day | Monday | Tuesday | Wednesday | Thursday | Friday | Comments |
| **Temperature** | | | | | | |
| **Fridge 1** | | | | | | |
| **Fridge2** | | | | | | |
| **Freezer 1** | | | | | | |
| **Freezer2** | | | | | | |
| | | | | | | |

# TEMPERATURE CONTROL LOG FORM

## General code of practice— Maintenance of Equipment

All equipments should be securely stored away in a locked cupboard.

All persons involve should know the correct procedure of cleaning and storage.

All equipments should be properly used for its designated task and properly cleaned after use and stored.

All equipments are inspected before and after use and all defects must be reported and logged.

All accompanied manufacturer's instructions must e followed during operations.

All electrical equipments must be maintained by authorised persons only.

# GENERAL CODE OF PRACTICE

## *Code of Practice for Extra Care Sheltered Housing*

The Code of Practice have ten standards; these must be met in order to achieve accreditation—to some, it is known as POVA (Protection of Vulnerable Adults) or QAF (Quality Framework Assessment), consisting of:

- Support Plans, Risk Assessments.
- Equality and Diversity.
- Security,
- Health and Safety.
- Confidentiality.
- Safeguarding.
- Complaints.
- Protection from Abuse.
- Professional Boundaries and Advocacy.
- Independence and Empowerment

The sheltered scheme manager should have knowledge of welfare benefits available to the tenants.

The sheltered scheme manager should be able to self motivate and able to supervise staff.

# REPAIRS

One very important task that every scheme manager does is to check and report repairs on behalf of the vulnerable tenant and also on behalf of the organisation in the communal areas as seemed fit (Health & Safety).

These reports are logged on two separate forms designed for record keeping.

These forms are sometimes referred to in times of doubts and disputes with the repairs office.

The first of these is known as the "TENANTS' FLAT REPAIRS" form as shown.

## TENANTS FLAT REPAIRS

| Date Reported | Flat No | Details of Repair | Ref. No. | Name of Contractor | Order of Urgency | Date Chased | Date Completed | Reported By |
|---|---|---|---|---|---|---|---|---|
|  |  |  |  |  |  |  |  |  |
|  |  |  |  |  |  |  |  |  |
|  |  |  |  |  |  |  |  |  |
|  |  |  |  |  |  |  |  |  |
|  |  |  |  |  |  |  |  |  |
|  |  |  |  |  |  |  |  |  |
|  |  |  |  |  |  |  |  |  |
|  |  |  |  |  |  |  |  |  |

The second form, known as "COMMUNAL AREA REPAIRS" form is shown below

| Date Reported | Details of Repair | Ref. No. | Order of Urgency | Name of Contractor | Date Chased | Date Repair completed | Reported By |
|---|---|---|---|---|---|---|---|
|  |  |  |  |  |  |  |  |
|  |  |  |  |  |  |  |  |
|  |  |  |  |  |  |  |  |
|  |  |  |  |  |  |  |  |
|  |  |  |  |  |  |  |  |
|  |  |  |  |  |  |  |  |
|  |  |  |  |  |  |  |  |

# MEDICATION ADMINISTRATION REPORT (MAR) SHEET

Medication Administration Record is known or called by the name MAR sheet.

Filling out Medication Administration Record (MAR) sheets is an important task that needs full attention.

This task is mainly seen happening in Extra Care sheltered housing or Care homes and in hospitals where the clients are usually prompted to take their medication.

The MAR sheet is used for recording how the medication is taken and it is supplied through the chemist/pharmacy.

Most care homes have the choice to choose which template best suit the kind of care that is being given and easy to use for their staff.

Most staff that prompts the clients to take their medication must attend training before hand.

This chart is a formal record of administration of medication within the extra care / care home or hospital and may be required for use as evidence in clinical investigations. It is therefore important that it is clear, accurate and up to date.

The MAR sheet is tailored to the person whose name appears on the sheet and reflects the items which are still being prescribed and administered.

## MEDICATION ADMINISTRATION REPORT (MAR) SHEET.

Name:................................  Address:................................  Doctor................................  Chemist................................

Start Date  (W/C ................)(W/C ................)(W/C ................)(W/C ................)(W/C ................)

| TIME | M T W Th F S Su | M T W Th F S Su | M T W Th F S Su | M T W Th F S Su |
|---|---|---|---|---|
| **PARACETAMOL TABLETS 500MG** **TAKE TWO AT NIGHT** | | | | |
| Breakfast | | | | |
| Lunch | | | | |
| Dinner | | | | |
| Evening | | | | |
| Dr sign      recd.      by | 2 | | | |

Key: R- refused, N- Nausea/vomiting, H – in hospital, D – destroyed, D/C-discontinued, W- withheld/other reason, A-away

| Name of Medication How to administer it | | | | |
|---|---|---|---|---|
| | | | | |
| Dr sign      recd.      by | 1 | | | |

Key: R- refused, N- Nausea/vomiting, H – in hospital, D – destroyed, D/C-discontinued, W- withheld/other reason, A-away

| | | | | |
|---|---|---|---|---|
| | | | | |
| Dr sign      recd.      by | | | | |

Key: R- refused, N- Nausea/vomiting, H – in hospital, D – destroyed, D/C-discontinued, W- withheld/other reason, A-away

| | | | | |
|---|---|---|---|---|
| | | | | |
| Dr sign      recd.      by | | | | |

Key: R- refused, N- Nausea/vomiting, H – in hospital, D – destroyed, D/C-discontinued, W- withheld/other reason, A-away

| | | | | |
|---|---|---|---|---|
| | | | | |
| Dr sign      recd.      by | | | | |

The MAR sheet must be printed clearly and contains the product name, strength, dose frequency, quantity, and any additional information required.

The MAR sheet includes a method that ensures any changes made after production are evident—dated, signed and indicates who has made the change.

The MAR sheet must be signed after each medication is administered and **NOT** before.

The completion of a MAR sheet must never be a guess or assumed work by the responsible staff.

# USEFUL INFORMATION

## Death of a Tenant

When someone dies in sheltered accommodation, what happens?

Especially if they had no-one living with them.

The tenancy will not end immediately after a tenant dies unless there is a written will from the late tenant; but if there is no written will, the only people who can end it are:-

## An Executor

This is someone named in a tenant's will as the person who will deal with the deceased possessions.

## An Administrator

This is someone who has applied to the Probate Registry and / or has the "Grant Probate"—letter of administration.

A Next of Kin, who is *NOT* one of the above, cannot end the tenancy after the death of a tenant.

## The Organisation's Legal Team

Where there is no Executor or Administrator, by law in any Council based sheltered accommodation, a Notice to Quit on the Public Trustee is served. This means that the tenancy will end in four /six weeks after the notice is served. During this time, if letters of Administration are obtained before the four /six weeks are up then the Administrator can end the tenancy.

A closing statement of the rent account will be sent to the person who will provide the deceased details for this purpose

# About the Author

V.K. Leigh is an experienced and practical sheltered scheme manager; having had the privilege of working with older persons in the United Kingdom; through some of the largest housing organisations; both in the private and public sectors.

Combining the gifts and years of practical experiences and his knowledge in sheltered housing, Extra Care and Mental Health; V.K.Leigh will undoubtedly be ranked as a professional in these sectors.

The writing of this book "**General Extra Care—*The Full Facts***" in sheltered housing sector of Supported Housing for the Vulnerable/Older Persons is knowledge being shared with anyone and everyone who reads or uses this book.

This book is a source of training manual, working book or as a literature to inform the intended staff that would want to work or interested in this sector; for knowledge.

V.K.Leigh continues to make researches into how to better the lifestyles and care for the older persons, searching for new ideas of how to further improve this field for all by providing trainings in modules.

V.K.Leigh is a professional business manager, consultant in management training, computer systems analyst, credit and financial analyst and member of some of the world's recognised professional bodies.

*—Other publications in Sheltered Housing by this author—*

1.  **General Guides to Management in Sheltered Housing**
2.  **Guides to Scheme Managers' operations**

www.ingramcontent.com/pod-product-compliance
Lightning Source LLC
Chambersburg PA
CBHW020400290526
45785CB00005B/2378